DIABETIC RENAL FOOD LIST

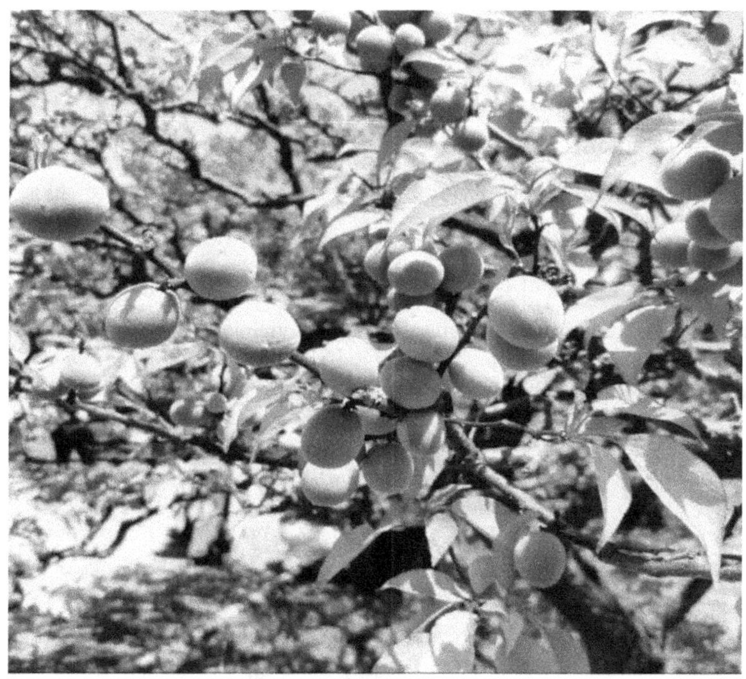

LORENE PEACHEY

DISCLAIMER

The content within this book reflects my thoughts, experiences, and beliefs. It is meant for informational and entertainment purposes. While I have taken great care to provide accurate information, I cannot guarantee the absolute correctness or applicability of the content to every individual or situation. Please consult with relevant professionals for advice specific to your needs.

TO GAIN ACCESS TO MORE BOOK BY THE AUTHOR SCAN THE QR CODE

TABLE OF CONTENTS

INTRODUCTION

In the realm of culinary exploration and nutritional alchemy, where the symphony of flavors meets the science of well-being, I am Nutrionist Lorene Peachey. It's not just a profession for me; it's a calling, a passion that has led me on a journey through the intricate corridors of dietary science. For over 25 years, I have immersed myself in the world of research, unraveling the secrets of optimal health, and crafting recipes that not only nourish the body but also ignite the taste buds.

My fascination with the interplay between food and health began long ago, fueled by a desire to make a meaningful impact on the lives of those grappling with the challenges of diabetes and renal health. This endeavor became my life's mission, prompting me to delve deep into the nuances of diabetic renal recipes, seeking a harmonious blend that transcends the mundane and transforms the therapeutic into the delightful.

As I stand at the crossroads of science and flavor, I am thrilled to share the fruits of my labor—a meticulously curated Diabetic Renal Food List. But before we embark on this culinary odyssey, let's ponder some questions that resonate with the soul.

Have you ever wondered about the stories that your food tells your body? Each morsel, a narrative woven into the very fabric of your well-being. What if your meals were not just sustenance but a symphony of healing, an art form that nurtures your body and elevates your spirit?

Picture this: a world where the food you consume becomes a vibrant tapestry of flavors, colors, and textures, carefully woven to address the unique needs of those managing diabetes and renal health. Imagine savoring each bite not just for its taste but for the transformative power it holds—a power to nourish, heal, and invigorate.

Now, let's traverse into the perilous territory of unhealthy eating. Close your eyes and envision the consequences of a diet devoid of mindfulness, a path where convenience trumps nutritional value. How does it feel to be ensnared in the clutches of processed foods, laden with sugars, sodium, and unhealthy fats? The heaviness in your gut, the lethargy in your limbs—these are the whispers of your body, yearning for a better, more nourishing path.

In my culinary journey, I've witnessed the aftermath of neglecting dietary needs. The silent struggle of those trapped in the quagmire of poor eating choices—the toll it takes on their bodies, their minds, and the very essence of their existence. It's a call to action, a plea to embrace the transformative potential of food as a catalyst for change.

Now, let's pivot to the realm of hope and possibility—a realm where a thoughtfully crafted Diabetic Renal Food List becomes a beacon of light. Imagine a resource that transcends the mundane boundaries of restriction, introducing you to a world of culinary wonders that not only align with dietary needs but also burst forth with flavor and vitality.

The benefits of embracing this curated food list are boundless. By weaving the principles of diabetes and renal health into every recipe, we unlock a treasure trove of advantages. Digest these thoughts: stabilized blood sugar levels, improved kidney function, increased energy levels, and a heightened sense of overall well-being. It's not just about what you eat; it's about reclaiming your life and savoring every moment.

With my 25 years of experience, I stand as a guide, a companion on your journey to wellness. Together, we traverse the landscape of tantalizing flavors and healthful choices. Picture a menu where succulent grilled salmon dances with zesty lemon-dill sauce, where vibrant quinoa bowls beckon with promises of nourishment, and where the humble cucumber transforms into a canvas for delectable tuna bites.

But let's not just talk about recipes; let's talk about stories—stories of rejuvenation, of individuals who took charge of their health and embarked on a culinary adventure. Imagine the joy of discovering a world where food is not just sustenance but a celebration—a celebration of life, health, and the extraordinary flavors that Mother Nature has bestowed upon us.

So, as we embark on this journey together, let the aroma of freshly prepared meals be the anthem of your vitality. Allow each bite to be a declaration—a declaration that you choose wellness, that you embrace the gift of health with open arms.

As I extend this Diabetic Renal Food List to you, it's not just a compilation of recipes; it's a testament to the transformative power of food. Let these recipes be your allies in the battle for better health, your companions in the pursuit of a life well-lived.

Join me on this culinary odyssey, where every recipe is a chapter in the book of your well-being—a book that you write with each mindful bite, with each exploration of flavors, and with each step toward a healthier, more vibrant you. The kitchen is our canvas, and the ingredients are our palette. Let the symphony of taste and health commence!

Contact the Author

Thank you for reading my book! I would love to hear from you, whether you have feedback, questions, or just want to share your thoughts. Your feedback means a lot to me and helps me improve as a writer.

Please don't hesitate to reach out to me through

lorenepeachey@gmail.com

I look forward to connecting with my readers and appreciate your support in this literary journey. Your thoughts and comments are valuable to me.

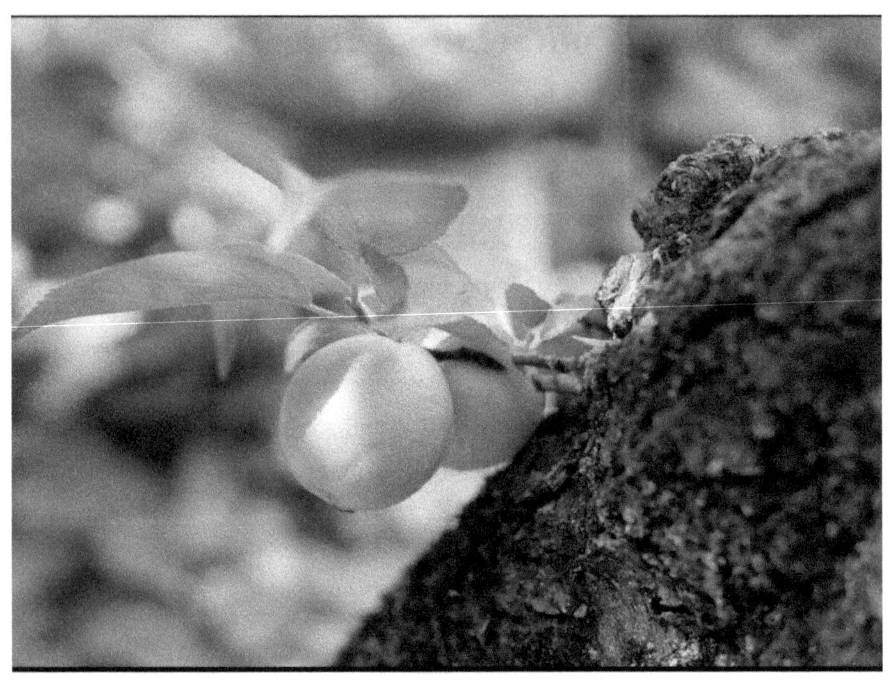

CHAPTER 1

UNDERSTANDING DIABETES

AND RENAL HEALTH

Diabetes and renal health are intricately connected, as individuals with diabetes are at an increased risk of developing kidney complications. The interplay between these two conditions necessitates a comprehensive understanding to effectively manage and improve overall well-being.

Diabetes

Diabetes is a chronic condition characterized by elevated blood sugar levels resulting from the body's inability to produce enough insulin or effectively use the insulin it produces. Over time, uncontrolled diabetes can lead to damage in various organs, including the kidneys.

Renal Implications of Diabetes

The kidneys play a vital role in filtering waste and excess fluids from the blood, regulating electrolytes, and maintaining a healthy balance in the body.

Diabetes can contribute to the development of diabetic kidney disease (nephropathy), a progressive condition that can ultimately lead to kidney failure if not managed appropriately.

The Importance of a Specialized Diet

Dietary choices have a profound impact on both diabetes management and renal health. A specialized diet tailored to the unique needs of individuals with diabetic renal conditions is crucial in mitigating the progression of kidney disease and maintaining stable blood sugar levels.

Key Considerations for a Diabetic Renal Diet

1. **Controlled Carbohydrate Intake:** Managing the quantity and quality of carbohydrates is essential for controlling blood sugar levels. Choosing complex carbohydrates with a low glycemic index can help prevent spikes in blood glucose.

2. **Limited Sodium Intake:** High blood pressure, common in diabetes, can exacerbate kidney damage. Therefore, reducing sodium intake is vital to managing blood pressure and preserving renal function.

3. **Moderate Protein Consumption:** Balancing protein intake is crucial, as excessive protein can strain the kidneys. Opting for lean protein sources and considering plant-based proteins can be beneficial.

4. **Phosphorus and Potassium Awareness:** Monitoring intake of phosphorus and potassium is important for individuals with compromised kidney function. Certain foods high in these minerals should be limited to prevent further stress on the kidneys.

5. **Hydration Management:** Adequate fluid intake is essential, but individuals with kidney complications may need to monitor their fluid intake more closely. Striking the right balance is key to preventing dehydration and overburdening the kidneys.

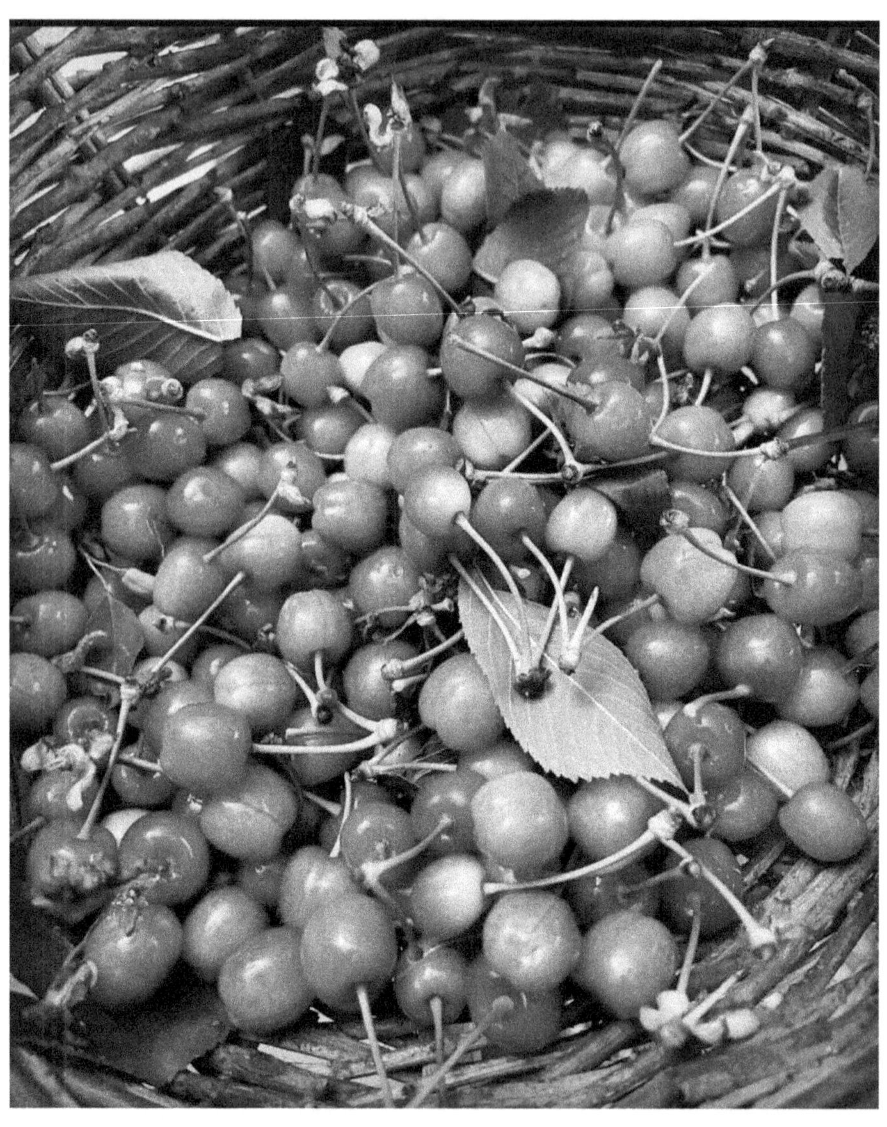

CHAPTER 2

BASICS OF DIABETIC RENAL DIET

Managing diabetes and renal health involves a balanced and thoughtful approach to dietary choices. The basics of a diabetic renal diet revolve around carefully balancing carbohydrates, proteins, and fats, while also keeping a close eye on blood sugar levels and managing fluid intake.

Balancing Carbohydrates, Proteins, and Fats

1. **Carbohydrates:**

   - Opt for complex carbohydrates with a low glycemic index to prevent rapid spikes in blood sugar levels.

   - Include whole grains, legumes, and vegetables in your diet for sustained energy release.

   - Practice portion control to manage overall carbohydrate intake throughout the day.

2. **Proteins:**

- Choose lean protein sources such as poultry, fish, tofu, and legumes to support muscle health.

- Monitor protein intake to avoid excessive strain on the kidneys. Consult with a healthcare professional to determine individualized protein requirements.

3. **Fats:**

- Prioritize healthy fats, such as those found in avocados, nuts, and olive oil.

- Limit saturated and trans fats to promote heart health.

- Be mindful of overall calorie intake from fats to maintain a healthy weight.

Monitoring Blood Sugar Levels:

1. **Regular Glucose Monitoring:**

- Establish a routine for monitoring blood sugar levels as advised by your healthcare provider.

- Keep a log of your readings to identify patterns and trends over time.

- Adjust your diet and medication as needed based on blood sugar level fluctuations.

2. **Meal Timing and Consistency:**

- Maintain a consistent eating schedule to help regulate blood sugar levels.

- Avoid skipping meals, and space your meals and snacks throughout the day to prevent extreme highs and lows in blood sugar.

3. **Understanding Glycemic Index:**

- Familiarize yourself with the glycemic index of foods to make informed choices that minimize blood sugar spikes.

- Include a variety of low-glycemic foods in your diet to promote stable blood sugar control.

Managing Fluid Intake

1. **Hydration Balance:**

- Stay adequately hydrated to support kidney function, but be mindful of fluid restrictions if advised by your healthcare team.

- Choose water as the primary beverage, and limit the intake of sugary drinks and high-sodium fluids.

2. **Monitoring Electrolytes:**

- Be aware of the potassium and phosphorus content in beverages, especially if managing renal complications.

- Consult with a healthcare professional to determine appropriate fluid and electrolyte goals.

3. **Individualized Recommendations:**

- Work closely with your healthcare team to establish personalized fluid intake goals based on your health status and kidney function.

CHAPTER 3

DIABETIC RENAL-FRIENDLY FOODS

Vegetables

1. **Cabbage:**

   - Nutritional Information (1 cup, raw):

     - Calories: 22

     - Carbohydrates: 5 grams

     - Protein: 1 gram

     - Fiber: 2 grams

     - Rich in vitamin C and a good source of fiber.

2. **Cauliflower:**

- Nutritional Information (1 cup, raw):

    - Calories: 27

    - Carbohydrates: 6 grams

    - Protein: 2 grams

    - Fiber: 3 grams

    - High in vitamin C and a good source of antioxidants.

3. **Bell Peppers (Assorted Colors):**

- Nutritional Information (1 cup, raw):

    - Calories: 46

    - Carbohydrates: 9 grams

    - Protein: 2 grams

    - Fiber: 3 grams

    - Rich in vitamins A and C, low in calories.

4. **Eggplant:**

- Nutritional Information (1 cup, cooked):

    - Calories: 35

    - Carbohydrates: 9 grams

    - Protein: 1 gram

    - Fiber: 3 grams

    - Low in calories, a source of antioxidants.

5. **Zucchini:**

- Nutritional Information (1 cup, raw):

    - Calories: 20

    - Carbohydrates: 4 grams

    - Protein: 1 gram

    - Fiber: 1 gram

    - Low-calorie option, source of vitamin C.

6. **Green Beans:**

- Nutritional Information (1 cup, raw):

    - Calories: 31

    - Carbohydrates: 7 grams

    - Protein: 2 grams

    - Fiber: 3 grams

    - Low in calories, a source of vitamin C.

7. **Kale:**

- Nutritional Information (1 cup, raw):

    - Calories: 33

    - Carbohydrates: 6 grams

    - Protein: 3 grams

    - Fiber: 1 gram

    - Packed with vitamins A, C, and K.

8. **Radishes:**

- Nutritional Information (1 cup, sliced):

  - Calories: 19

  - Carbohydrates: 4 grams

  - Protein: 1 gram

  - Fiber: 2 grams

  - Low in calories and a source of vitamin C.

9. **Summer Squash:**

- Nutritional Information (1 cup, sliced):

  - Calories: 20

  - Carbohydrates: 5 grams

  - Protein: 1 gram

  - Fiber: 2 grams

  - Low in calories, a source of vitamin C.

10. **Turnips:**

- Nutritional Information (1 cup, cooked):

  - Calories: 51

  - Carbohydrates: 12 grams

  - Protein: 2 grams

  - Fiber: 3 grams

  - Good source of vitamin C and fiber.

Fruits

1. **Berries (e.g., Strawberries):**

    - Nutritional Information (1 cup, whole):

        - Calories: 49

        - Carbohydrates: 12 grams

        - Fiber: 3 grams

        - Vitamin C: 89 mg

        - Antioxidant-rich, low in sugar.

2. **Apples:**

    - Nutritional Information (1 medium-sized apple):

        - Calories: 95

        - Carbohydrates: 25 grams

        - Fiber: 4 grams

        - Vitamin C: 14% DV

        - Contains soluble fiber, aiding digestion.

3. **Pears:**

- Nutritional Information (1 medium-sized pear):

    - Calories: 101

    - Carbohydrates: 27 grams

    - Fiber: 6 grams

    - Vitamin C: 7% DV

    - Provides dietary fiber and natural sweetness.

4. **Cherries:**

- Nutritional Information (1 cup, pitted):

    - Calories: 87

    - Carbohydrates: 22 grams

    - Fiber: 3 grams

    - Vitamin C: 16% DV

    - Rich in antioxidants, lower in sugar.

5. **Peaches:**

- Nutritional Information (1 medium-sized peach):

    - Calories: 59

    - Carbohydrates: 14 grams

    - Fiber: 2 grams

    - Vitamin C: 10% DV

    - Low in calories and a good source of vitamins.

6. **Plums:**

- Nutritional Information (2 medium-sized plums):

    - Calories: 60

    - Carbohydrates: 16 grams

    - Fiber: 2 grams

    - Vitamin C: 16% DV

    - Low in calories and a source of antioxidants.

7. **Apricots:**

- Nutritional Information (3 medium-sized apricots):

    - Calories: 50

    - Carbohydrates: 12 grams

    - Fiber: 2 grams

    - Vitamin C: 10% DV

    - Contains beta-carotene and fiber.

8. **Watermelon:**

- Nutritional Information (1 cup, diced):

    - Calories: 46

    - Carbohydrates: 12 grams

    - Fiber: 1 gram

    - Vitamin C: 13% DV

    - Hydrating and low in calories.

9. **Grapes:**

- Nutritional Information (1 cup, seedless):

    - Calories: 104

    - Carbohydrates: 27 grams

    - Fiber: 1 gram

    - Vitamin C: 27% DV

    - Contains natural sugars, consume in moderation.

10. **Kiwi:**

- Nutritional Information (1 medium-sized kiwi):

    - Calories: 50

    - Carbohydrates: 13 grams

    - Fiber: 2.5 grams

    - Vitamin C: 71% DV

    - High in vitamin C and dietary fiber.

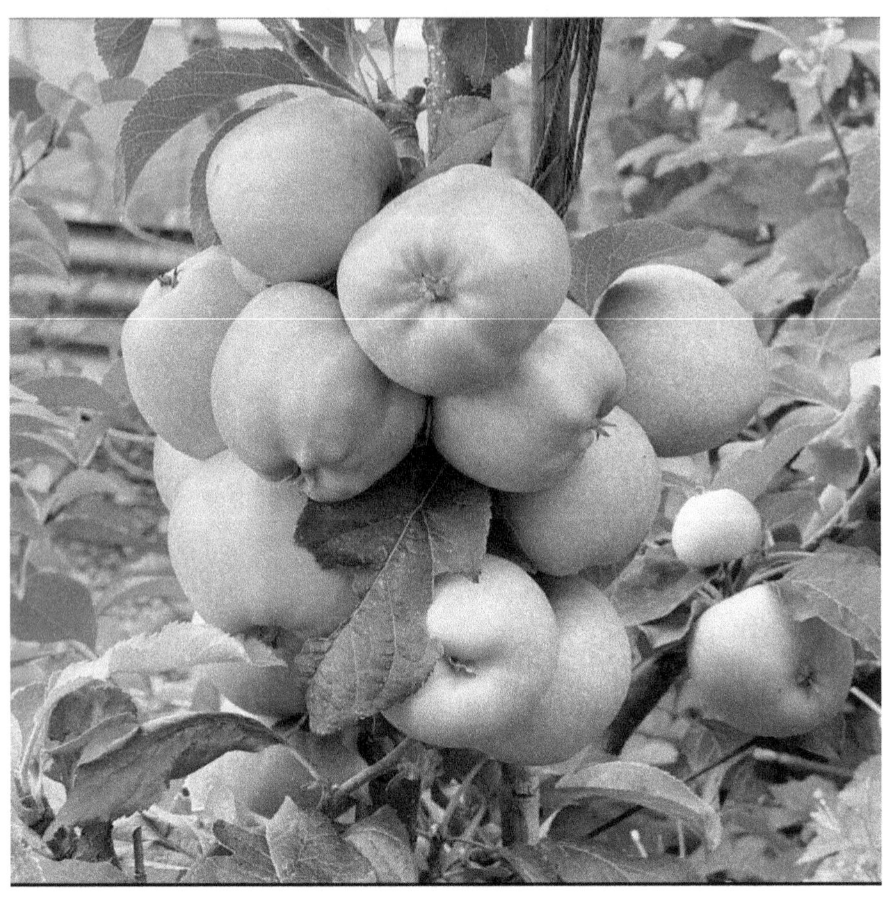

Lean Proteins

1. **Chicken Breast (Skinless, Grilled):**

   - Nutritional Information (3 ounces):

     - Calories: 128

     - Protein: 26 grams

     - Fat: 3 grams

     - Saturated Fat: 1 gram

     - Low in fat, high in protein.

2. **Turkey (Ground, 93% Lean, Cooked):**

   - Nutritional Information (3 ounces):

     - Calories: 176

     - Protein: 22 grams

     - Fat: 9 grams

     - Saturated Fat: 2.5 grams

     - Lean source of protein.

3. **Fish (Salmon, Baked or Grilled):**

- Nutritional Information (3 ounces):

    - Calories: 155

    - Protein: 22 grams

    - Fat: 7 grams

    - Omega-3 Fatty Acids: 1.8 grams

    - Heart-healthy fats and high-quality protein.

4. **Tofu:**

- Nutritional Information (1/2 cup, firm):

    - Calories: 94

    - Protein: 10 grams

    - Fat: 6 grams

    - Saturated Fat: 0.8 grams

    - Plant-based protein source.

5. **Egg Whites (Boiled):**

- Nutritional Information (3 large egg whites):

    - Calories: 51

    - Protein: 11 grams

    - Fat: 0 grams

    - Cholesterol: 0 mg

    - Low in calories and fat, cholesterol-free.

6. **Lean Beef (Sirloin, Grilled):**

- Nutritional Information (3 ounces):

    - Calories: 160

    - Protein: 26 grams

    - Fat: 5 grams

    - Saturated Fat: 2 grams

    - Moderately lean choice.

7. **Pork Tenderloin (Roasted):**

- Nutritional Information (3 ounces):

    - Calories: 143

    - Protein: 24 grams

    - Fat: 4 grams

    - Saturated Fat: 1 gram

    - Lean cut of pork.

8. **Chicken Thighs (Skinless, Baked):**

- Nutritional Information (3 ounces):

    - Calories: 166

    - Protein: 19 grams

    - Fat: 10 grams

    - Saturated Fat: 2.5 grams

    - Moderation is key due to slightly higher fat content.

9. **Shrimp (Boiled or Grilled):**

- Nutritional Information (3 ounces):

  - Calories: 84

  - Protein: 18 grams

  - Fat: 1 gram

  - Low in calories, high in protein.

10. **Cottage Cheese (Low-Fat):**

- Nutritional Information (1/2 cup):

  - Calories: 80

  - Protein: 14 grams

  - Fat: 2 grams

  - Saturated Fat: 1 gram

  - Source of protein with lower fat content.

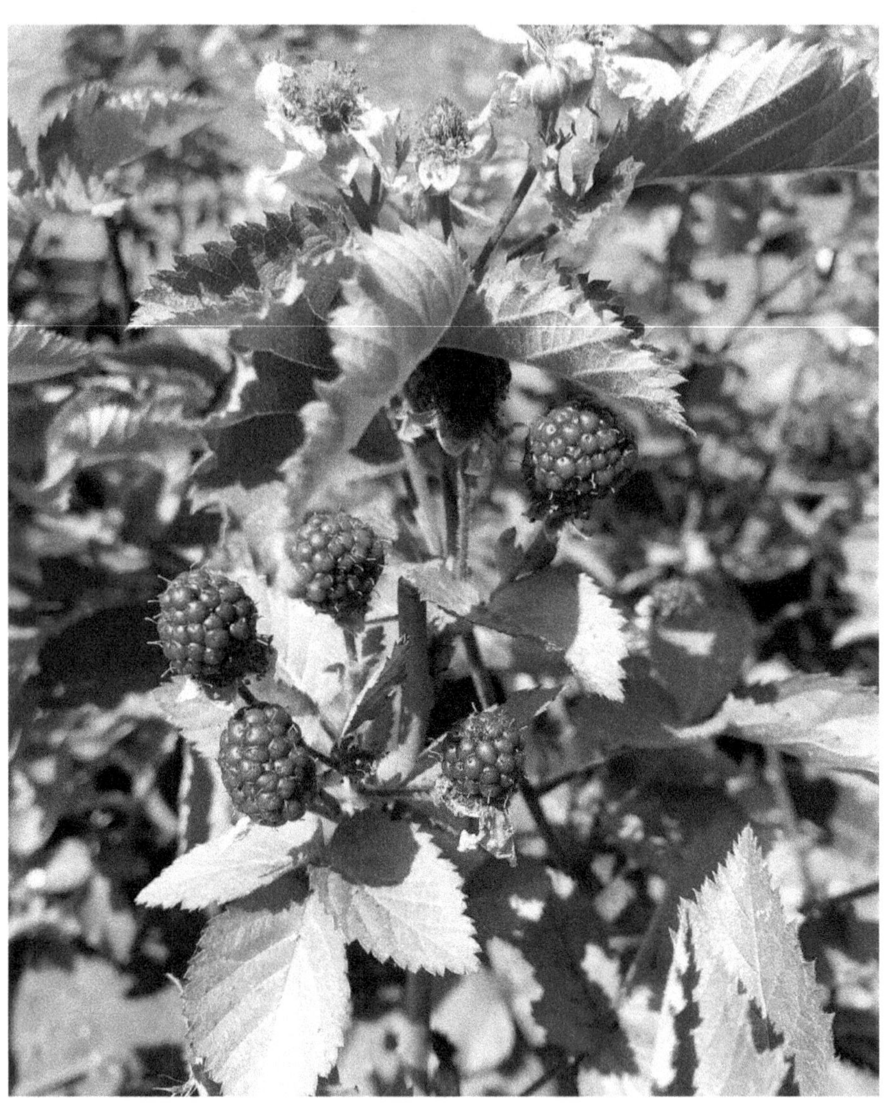

CHAPTER 4

FOODS TO LIMIT OR AVOID

1. **Processed Meats (e.g., Hot Dogs, Sausages):**

   - Nutritional Information (1 serving):

     - High in sodium, often containing more than 500 mg per serving.

     - Processed meats may also have added preservatives and unhealthy fats.

2. **Canned Soups and Broths:**

   - Nutritional Information (1 cup):

     - Extremely high in sodium, with some varieties exceeding 800 mg per cup.

     - Increased sodium intake can negatively impact blood pressure and kidney health.

3. **Fast Food Burgers and Fries:**

- Nutritional Information (Typical serving):

    - High in saturated fats, trans fats, and sodium.

    - Can contribute to weight gain and negatively affect cardiovascular health.

4. **Sugary Beverages (e.g., Soda, Sweetened Iced Tea):**

- Nutritional Information (12 ounces):

    - Loaded with added sugars, contributing to elevated blood glucose levels.

    - Can lead to dehydration and increased calorie intake.

5. **Packaged Snack Foods (e.g., Potato Chips, Pretzels):**

- Nutritional Information (Typical serving):

    - High in sodium, often exceeding 200 mg per serving.

    - May contain unhealthy fats contributing to inflammation and kidney strain.

6. **Certain Fruits High in Potassium (e.g., Bananas):**

   - Nutritional Information (1 medium-sized banana):

      - High in potassium, which can be problematic for individuals with compromised kidney function.

      - While nutritious, moderation is advised.

7. **High-Potassium Vegetables (e.g., Potatoes, Sweet Potatoes):**

   - Nutritional Information (1 medium-sized potato):

      - Potatoes are rich in potassium, and excessive intake can be challenging for renal health.

      - Limiting portion size is recommended.

8. **Whole Grain Products with Added Sugars:**

   - Nutritional Information (Varies by product):

      - Some whole grain products may contain added sugars, impacting blood sugar levels.

      - Choose whole grains without added sugars when possible.

9. **Desserts and Pastries:**

- Nutritional Information (Varies by dessert):

    - Often high in sugar, unhealthy fats, and refined carbohydrates.

    - Can contribute to spikes in blood sugar and may exacerbate kidney issues.

10. **High-Potassium Dairy Products (e.g., Whole Milk, Yogurt):**

- Nutritional Information (Varies by product):

    - Dairy products can be high in potassium, which may need to be limited in a renal diet.

    - Opt for lower-potassium dairy alternatives or consult with a dietitian.

CHAPTER 5

RECIPES FOR DIABETIC RENAL DIETS

Breakfast Ideas

Veggie Omelette

Cooking Time: 10 minutes

Servings: 2

Ingredients:

- 4 large eggs

- 1/4 cup diced bell peppers

- 1/4 cup diced tomatoes

- 1/4 cup chopped spinach

- Salt and pepper to taste

- 1 tablespoon olive oil

Instructions:

1. Whisk eggs in a bowl and season with salt and pepper.

2. Heat olive oil in a non-stick pan over medium heat.

3. Add veggies to the pan and sauté until slightly tender.

4. Pour whisked eggs over the veggies, cook until edges set, then flip to cook the other side.

5. Once cooked through, fold the omelette, and serve.

Nutritional Information:

Per Serving - Calories: 180, Protein: 14g, Carbohydrates: 4g, Fat: 12g

Greek Yogurt Parfait

Preparation Time: 5 minutes

Servings: 1

Ingredients:

- 1/2 cup Greek yogurt (low-fat)

- 1/4 cup fresh berries (e.g., blueberries, strawberries)

- 2 tablespoons chopped nuts (e.g., almonds, walnuts)

- 1 teaspoon honey or a sugar substitute

Instructions:

1. In a glass or bowl, layer Greek yogurt.

2. Add a layer of fresh berries and chopped nuts.

3. Drizzle honey or use a sugar substitute.

4. Repeat layers as desired.

5. Serve immediately.

Nutritional Information:

Per Serving - Calories: 220, Protein: 15g, Carbohydrates: 18g, Fat: 10g

Quinoa Breakfast Bowl

Cooking Time: 15 minutes

Servings: 2

Ingredients:

- 1 cup cooked quinoa

- 1/2 cup sliced strawberries

- 1/4 cup sliced bananas

- 2 tablespoons chopped almonds

- 1 tablespoon chia seeds

- 1/2 cup unsweetened almond milk

Instructions:

1. Divide cooked quinoa into two bowls.

2. Top with sliced strawberries, bananas, chopped almonds, and chia seeds.

3. Pour almond milk over the bowl.

4. Mix ingredients and enjoy.

Nutritional Information:

Per Serving - Calories: 280, Protein: 8g, Carbohydrates: 35g, Fat: 12g

Cottage Cheese and Berry Bowl

Preparation Time: 5 minutes

Servings: 1

Ingredients:

- 1/2 cup low-fat cottage cheese

- 1/2 cup mixed berries (e.g., blueberries, raspberries)

- 1 tablespoon chopped nuts (e.g., walnuts, almonds)

- 1 teaspoon chia seeds

- 1 teaspoon honey or a sugar substitute

Instructions:

1. In a bowl, combine cottage cheese and mixed berries.

2. Top with chopped nuts, chia seeds, and drizzle with honey or use a sugar substitute.

3. Mix well and enjoy.

Nutritional Information:

Per Serving - Calories: 220, Protein: 15g, Carbohydrates: 20g, Fat: 10g

Chia Seed Pudding

Preparation Time: 5 minutes (plus chilling time)

Servings: 2

Ingredients:

- 1/4 cup chia seeds
- 1 cup unsweetened almond milk
- 1/2 teaspoon vanilla extract
- 1 tablespoon chopped nuts (e.g., pistachios, almonds)
- Fresh berries for topping

Instructions:

1. In a bowl, mix chia seeds, almond milk, and vanilla extract.
2. Refrigerate for at least 2 hours or overnight until it thickens.
3. Stir well before serving.
4. Top with chopped nuts and fresh berries.

Nutritional Information:

Per Serving - Calories: 150, Protein: 5g, Carbohydrates: 12g, Fat: 9g

Lunch and Dinner Recipes

Grilled Salmon with Lemon-Dill Sauce

Cooking Time: 15 minutes

Servings: 2

Ingredients:

- 2 salmon fillets (6 ounces each)

- 1 tablespoon olive oil

- 1 teaspoon lemon zest

- 1 tablespoon fresh lemon juice

- 1 tablespoon fresh dill, chopped

- Salt and pepper to taste

Instructions:

1. Preheat the grill.

2. Rub salmon fillets with olive oil and season with salt and pepper.

3. Grill salmon for 6-8 minutes per side, or until cooked through.

4. In a small bowl, mix lemon zest, lemon juice, and chopped dill to make the sauce.

5. Drizzle the lemon-dill sauce over grilled salmon and serve.

Nutritional Information:

Per Serving - Calories: 320, Protein: 36g, Carbohydrates: 1g, Fat: 19g

Quinoa and Vegetable Stir-Fry

Cooking Time: 20 minutes

Servings: 4

Ingredients:

- 1 cup quinoa, cooked

- 1 tablespoon vegetable oil

- 1 cup broccoli florets

- 1 bell pepper, sliced

- 1 carrot, julienned

- 1 cup snow peas

- 2 cloves garlic, minced

- 2 tablespoons low-sodium soy sauce

Instructions:

1. Heat oil in a wok or skillet over medium-high heat.

2. Add garlic, broccoli, bell pepper, carrot, and snow peas. Stir-fry for 5-7 minutes.

3. Add cooked quinoa and soy sauce. Toss until well combined.

4. Cook for an additional 2-3 minutes, ensuring even heating.

5. Serve hot.

Nutritional Information:

Per Serving - Calories: 220, Protein: 8g, Carbohydrates: 35g, Fat: 6g

Chicken and Vegetable Skewers

Cooking Time: 20 minutes (plus marinating time)
Servings: 3

Ingredients:

- 1 pound chicken breast, cut into cubes

- 1 zucchini, sliced

- 1 bell pepper, cut into chunks

- 1 red onion, cut into wedges

- 2 tablespoons olive oil

- 1 teaspoon dried oregano

- 1 teaspoon garlic powder

- Salt and pepper to taste

Instructions:

1. In a bowl, combine olive oil, dried oregano, garlic powder, salt, and pepper.

2. Add chicken cubes to the marinade and refrigerate for at least 30 minutes.

3. Preheat the grill.

4. Thread marinated chicken and vegetables onto skewers.

5. Grill for 10-12 minutes, turning occasionally, until chicken is fully cooked.

6. Serve hot.

Nutritional Information:

Per Serving - Calories: 290, Protein: 25g, Carbohydrates: 10g, Fat: 16g

Lentil and Vegetable Soup

Cooking Time: 30 minutes

Servings: 6

Ingredients:

- 1 cup dry green lentils, rinsed

- 1 onion, diced

- 2 carrots, chopped

- 2 celery stalks, chopped

- 2 cloves garlic, minced

- 1 can (14 oz) diced tomatoes

- 6 cups low-sodium vegetable broth

- 1 teaspoon ground cumin

- 1 teaspoon smoked paprika

- Salt and pepper to taste

Instructions:

1. In a large pot, sauté onions, carrots, and celery until softened.

2. Add minced garlic and cook for an additional minute.

3. Add lentils, diced tomatoes, vegetable broth, cumin, smoked paprika, salt, and pepper.

4. Bring to a boil, then reduce heat and simmer for 20-25 minutes or until lentils are tender.

5. Adjust seasoning and serve hot.

Nutritional Information:

Per Serving - Calories: 220, Protein: 13g, Carbohydrates: 38g, Fat: 1g

Baked Cod with Roasted Vegetables

Cooking Time: 25 minutes

Servings: 2

Ingredients:

- 2 cod fillets (6 ounces each)

- 1 cup cherry tomatoes, halved

- 1 zucchini, sliced

- 1 yellow bell pepper, sliced

- 2 tablespoons olive oil

- 1 teaspoon dried thyme

- 1 teaspoon lemon zest

- Salt and pepper to taste

Instructions:

1. Preheat the oven to 400°F (200°C).

2. Place cod fillets on a baking sheet.

3. In a bowl, toss cherry tomatoes, zucchini, and yellow bell pepper with olive oil, thyme, lemon zest, salt, and pepper.

4. Spread the vegetable mixture around the cod fillets on the baking sheet.

5. Bake for 15-20 minutes or until the fish is opaque and flakes easily.

6. Serve hot.

Nutritional Information:

Per Serving - Calories: 290, Protein: 30g, Carbohydrates: 12g, Fat: 15g

Desserts and Snacks

Berry Yogurt Parfait

Preparation Time: 10 minutes

Servings: 2

Ingredients:

- 1 cup Greek yogurt (low-fat)
- 1/2 cup mixed berries (e.g., blueberries, strawberries)
- 2 tablespoons chopped nuts (e.g., almonds, walnuts)
- 1 teaspoon chia seeds
- 1 teaspoon honey or a sugar substitute

Instructions:

1. In a glass or bowl, layer Greek yogurt.
2. Add a layer of mixed berries and chopped nuts.
3. Sprinkle chia seeds over the layers.
4. Drizzle honey or use a sugar substitute.
5. Repeat layers as desired.

Nutritional Information:

Per Serving - Calories: 220, Protein: 15g, Carbohydrates: 20g, Fat: 10g

Baked Apple with Cinnamon

Cooking Time: 30 minutes

Servings: 2

Ingredients:

- 2 medium-sized apples, cored and halved
- 1 tablespoon unsalted butter, melted
- 1 teaspoon ground cinnamon
- 1 tablespoon chopped nuts (e.g., pecans, almonds)
- 1 teaspoon honey or a sugar substitute

Instructions:

1. Preheat the oven to 375°F (190°C).
2. Place apple halves in a baking dish.
3. Mix melted butter and cinnamon, then brush over the apples.
4. Bake for 25-30 minutes or until apples are tender.
5. Sprinkle chopped nuts and drizzle honey or use a sugar substitute.

Nutritional Information:

Per Serving - Calories: 160, Protein: 1g, Carbohydrates: 30g, Fat: 6g

Chia Seed Pudding with Berries

Preparation Time: 5 minutes (plus chilling time)

Servings: 2

Ingredients:

- 1/4 cup chia seeds

- 1 cup unsweetened almond milk

- 1/2 teaspoon vanilla extract

- 1 tablespoon chopped nuts (e.g., pistachios, almonds)

- 1/2 cup mixed berries for topping

Instructions:

1. In a bowl, mix chia seeds, almond milk, and vanilla extract.

2. Refrigerate for at least 2 hours or overnight until it thickens.

3. Stir well before serving.

4. Top with chopped nuts and mixed berries.

Nutritional Information:

Per Serving - Calories: 150, Protein: 5g, Carbohydrates: 12g, Fat: 9g

Cucumber and Tuna Bites

Preparation Time: 10 minutes

Servings: 2

Ingredients:

- 1 cucumber, sliced into rounds

- 1 can (5 ounces) tuna, drained

- 1 tablespoon Greek yogurt (low-fat)

- 1 teaspoon Dijon mustard

- Fresh dill for garnish

- Salt and pepper to taste

Instructions:

1. In a bowl, mix tuna, Greek yogurt, Dijon mustard, salt, and pepper.

2. Place a dollop of the tuna mixture on each cucumber round.

3. Garnish with fresh dill.

4. Serve chilled.

Nutritional Information:

Per Serving - Calories: 140, Protein: 18g, Carbohydrates: 3g, Fat: 6g

Baked Cinnamon-Spiced Pears

Cooking Time: 20 minutes

Servings: 2

Ingredients:

- 2 ripe but firm pears, halved and cored
- 1 tablespoon melted butter
- 1 teaspoon ground cinnamon
- 1 tablespoon chopped walnuts
- 1 teaspoon honey or a sugar substitute

Instructions:

1. Preheat the oven to 375°F (190°C).
2. Place pear halves in a baking dish.
3. Mix melted butter and cinnamon, then brush over the pears.
4. Sprinkle chopped walnuts on top.
5. Bake for 15-20 minutes or until pears are tender.
6. Drizzle honey or use a sugar substitute before serving.

Nutritional Information:

Per Serving - Calories: 180, Protein: 2g, Carbohydrates: 30g, Fat: 8g

IF YOU WANT MORE RECIPES, YOU CAN CHECK OUT OTHER BOOKS BY THE AUTHOR

DIABETIC RENAL DIET COOKBOOK FOR NEWLY DAIGNOSED

RENAL DIET COOKBOOK FOR NEWLY DIAGNOSED

RENAL DIET COOKBOOK FOR SENIORS

RENAL DIET AIR FRYER COOKBOOK FOR SENIORS

KIDNEY DIEASE COOKBOOK FOR WOMEN

TO GET ACCESS TO MORE BOOKS BY THE AUTHOR SCAN THE QR CODE

CONCLUSION

As we reach the final chapter of our culinary journey through the world of Diabetic Renal Food, I want to express my deepest gratitude for accompanying me on this adventure. It has been a pleasure to share my passion for nutrition and wellness with you, weaving together the threads of science and flavor to create a tapestry of healthful and delicious possibilities.

In our exploration, we've uncovered the transformative potential of mindful eating, where each ingredient serves a purpose, and each recipe is a step toward a healthier, more vibrant life. The Diabetic Renal Food List is not just a compilation of dishes; it is a testament to the extraordinary synergy between nourishment and delight—a fusion that extends beyond the confines of dietary restrictions to embrace a life of culinary joy.

As you embark on your own culinary exploration, I invite you to savor the flavors, relish the textures, and celebrate the healing potential of every meal. Each recipe is an opportunity to nurture your body, support your well-being, and revel in the pleasure of mindful eating.

Your feedback is invaluable to me. I encourage you to share your thoughts, experiences, and any creative twists you bring to these recipes. Let this journey be a dialogue—a conversation about the joys, challenges, and triumphs of embracing a healthful and flavorful lifestyle.

If you discover a new variation, a substitution that elevates a dish, or simply want to share the impact these recipes have had on your well-being, I'm eager to hear from you. Your insights can inspire others on their journey to wellness, creating a community bound by a shared commitment to health and culinary enjoyment.

Together, let's continue to explore the boundless possibilities that food offers for nurturing our bodies and delighting our senses. Thank you for being a part of this enriching experience, and I look forward to hearing from you as we continue this journey toward a healthier, happier, and more flavorful life.

Bon appétit, and may your culinary adventures be filled with vitality and joy!

BONUS CHAPTER

LIFESTYLE AND EXERCISE TIPS

Maintaining an active lifestyle is crucial for individuals managing diabetes and renal health. Regular physical activity offers numerous benefits, including improved blood sugar control, cardiovascular health, and overall well-being. Here are some key recommendations:

1. **Aerobic Exercise:**

   - Engage in moderate-intensity aerobic exercise such as brisk walking, cycling, or swimming for at least 150 minutes per week.

   - Aim for at least 75 minutes of vigorous-intensity aerobic exercise if preferred, spread throughout the week.

2. **Strength Training:**

   - Include strength training exercises at least two days a week.

   - Focus on major muscle groups using resistance bands, weights, or bodyweight exercises.

3. **Flexibility and Balance:**

- Incorporate flexibility exercises such as stretching and yoga to enhance joint mobility.

- Include balance exercises to reduce the risk of falls, especially for individuals with kidney issues.

4. **Consistency is Key:**

- Aim for regularity in physical activity, spreading sessions across the week to maintain overall health.

- Gradually increase intensity and duration to challenge the body positively.

5. **Consultation with Healthcare Professionals:**

- Individuals with diabetes and renal concerns should consult healthcare providers before starting a new exercise regimen.

- Tailor exercise plans based on individual health conditions and capabilities.

Stress Management for Diabetes and Renal Health

Managing stress is essential for individuals dealing with diabetes and renal concerns. Chronic stress can adversely affect blood sugar levels and overall health. Incorporating stress management techniques into daily life is crucial:

1. **Mindfulness and Meditation:**

   - Practice mindfulness and meditation techniques to promote relaxation and reduce stress.

   - Mindful breathing exercises and guided meditation can be effective tools.

2. **Regular Exercise:**

   - Engage in regular physical activity, as exercise is a powerful stress reliever.

   - Choose activities that bring joy and can be sustained over time.

3. **Healthy Sleep Habits:**

   - Prioritize quality sleep by maintaining a consistent sleep schedule.

- Create a relaxing bedtime routine to improve the overall sleep experience.

4. **Social Connections:**

    - Foster supportive relationships with family and friends.

    - Share feelings and concerns to alleviate emotional burdens.

5. **Time Management:**

    - Organize daily tasks and prioritize responsibilities.

    - Break down larger tasks into manageable steps to reduce feelings of overwhelm.

6. **Professional Support:**

    - Seek guidance from mental health professionals or support groups to manage stress effectively.

    - Addressing emotional well-being is integral to comprehensive diabetes and renal care.

7. **Hobbies and Enjoyable Activities:**

- Dedicate time to hobbies and activities that bring joy and relaxation.

- Balancing work and leisure contributes to overall mental well-being

BONUS EMAIL CONSULTATION

Embark on a transformative wellness journey with a bonus free email consultation led by a seasoned nutritionist boasting 25 years of expertise. This exclusive opportunity invites you to delve into a personalized chapter of health, where I will share invaluable insights and tailored advice to elevate your overall well-being. Whether you seek weight management, nutritional guidance, or specific health improvements, my wealth of experience ensures a comprehensive approach to meet your unique needs.

During this consultation, we will explore your current lifestyle, dietary preferences, and wellness aspirations. By collaborating through email, I aim to provide you with a roadmap for sustainable health and vitality. Seize this chance to ask questions, address concerns, and gain a deeper understanding of how nutrition can positively impact your life. To claim your bonus chapter consultation, simply send me an email with a brief overview of your health goals, and let's kickstart your journey to a healthier, more vibrant you.

lorenepeachey@gmail.com